Vegan Keto

Eat right, not less

By:

Holly R.Evans

About This Book

As many people get to know about keto diet, it is becoming increasingly clear that there is no single "right" approach to accomplish and maintain ketosis. Many popular voices in the keto space offer a perspective that differs from the traditional, more dogmatic approach to low-carb eating. It has been really cool to watch the popularity of this diet grow over the years and to see the different tips, strategies, and even products that members of the keto community think of. This book serves as an excellent guide on how to follow a Vegan Keto diet and lifestyle.

This book will provide you with:
All what you need to succeed with the Vegan Keto:

- Simple cooking ideas, safe and non-demanding weight loss strategy,
- Adopt healthy habits
- Achieve long-term success

TABLE OF CONTENTS

INTRODUCTION

A ketogenic diet refers to one that is low in carbohydrates, which will allow the body to break down fat faster in order to metabolize ketones.
It's also the inclusion of real food and wholesome ingredients. Besides, a vegetarian binging on donuts, fries, and cheese is doing their health and environment a disservice as much as any other food junkie.

Are you anxious to lose some unwanted pounds and looking for something that can burn fat at maximum speed? Have you tried endless other diet plans but didn't work for more than a few weeks?
This book is mainly for you.

WAY TO ACHIEVE MAINTAIN KETOSIS

We will explore what you need to know about ketosis

KETOSIS – WHAT DOES IT MEAN?

In the simplest terms, it is a state achieved when fat burning is active. The body starts burning fat and its proteins, in exchange for energy. We can talk about the state of ketosis when the concentration of glucose is lesser than that of the level of ketone bodies in the blood. The ketogenic diet is a low carbohydrate diet.

FASTER FAT BURNING

The body of each of us has an unwanted fat. Thanks to ketosis it is easy to get rid of it because the body burns fat tissue. Eating carbohydrates, the body first consumes glycogen stores (energy reserve used for physical activity), then fat. It is, therefore, a much longer process. If you do not eat carbohydrates, there is no glucose in your blood, so you ask where the energy is being taken from? The body, instead of insulin, starts glucagon at the moment, which is what breaks down the fat tissue - as it can not use sugars because we did not provide them. Energy, in this case, arises from the burning of fat stores.

SMALLER APPETITE

Ketone bodies, formed by decomposition of fats, limit hunger. Often, despite the small portion, the meal is high in calories due to its fat content. By excluding carbohydrates from your diet, you limit insulin fluctuations and hunger pangs caused by them.

HOW TO START?

It is best to take small steps to avoid feeling unwell and stomach problems that can occur with a drastic change in diet and sudden carbohydrate trimming. Initially, you can start with consuming 25-30% carbohydrates, 40% protein 35% fat. Then, observing the effects, we reduce carbohydrates by 5% to obtain a supply of 50-80 g of carbs a day.

The best way to enter the state of ketosis is a large intake of fats with a small amount of protein, and you can also eat about 50 grams of carbohydrates a day.

WHAT FATS CAN YOU USE?

Diversifying sources of fat is essential. It can not be based, for example, only on animal fats. Eat also fatty fish, olive oil, coconut oil, avocado, nuts, seeds and seeds.

How to function since carbohydrates are the source of the fastest assimilable energy, and glucose, which is processed after the body consumes them, is energy for the brain.
It is thanks to the abundant supply of fat that the body can produce ketone bodies that provide energy and food also for the brain.

Let's go back to our ancestors who did not know cereals, fruits or vegetables. Their primary source of energy was fats.

Now the question is, what about carbohydrates? Eat or not eat?

Follow and listen to your body! Personally, as an athlete, I do not recommend completely giving up carbohydrates, especially to active people. I am the most like this when it comes to carbohydrate intake after training.

Remember that if the active person's diet is low in carbohydrates, symptoms such as irritability, tiredness, sleep disturbances, loss of joy of life, and frustrations may occur. This will mean that the adrenal glands that are depleted with low sugar levels excessively produce cortisol. There will be a problem with obtaining glucose and creating energy by eliminating carbohydrates. Exhaustion of the adrenal glands causes difficulty in the conversion of glycogen. Then the thyroid slows down, the body is still cold, there is no desire for sex, you do not know when you are full and when you do not, you have a sweet, disturbed sleep, stop menstruating, gain weight.

And you need 50 - 70 g of carbohydrates a day to maintain a relative balance. I'm not talking about overeating bread or cereals in general. Remember that carbohydrates are also found in vegetables - potatoes, sweet potatoes, root vegetables or pumpkin.

If your daily energy expenditure does not require a large supply of carbohydrates, put on protein-fat meals, especially in the morning. Carbohydrate eats for a second breakfast. My observations confirm: if you want to significantly reduce carbohydrates and not lose health, then you need to increase the amount of fat in the diet.

Fat along with the protein give a significant signal of satiety but on the condition that you eat slowly and thoroughly biting. Such meals have a smaller volume than carbohydrates, and sometimes we eat more than we should, to feel full.

In case you care about the increase in muscle mass, it even requires increasing the amount of coals in the diet.

The ketogenic diet is not the best option for people with liver, pancreas or kidney problems. Managing a greater burden due to the metabolism of ketones will be a problem.

WHOM IS KETOGENIC DIET REALLY GOOD FOR?

For people with autoimmune diseases, with diabetes, insulin-resistant. Also for some cancers, for problems with the intestines like FODMAPS, issues with the absorption of sugars and fibre.

An example of a one-day menu proposed by me:
This is an sample of a one-day meal for an athlete

On an empty stomach:
 Protein (e.g., immunocal)

Breakfast:
Quinoa with sour fruits such as pomegranate and raspberries

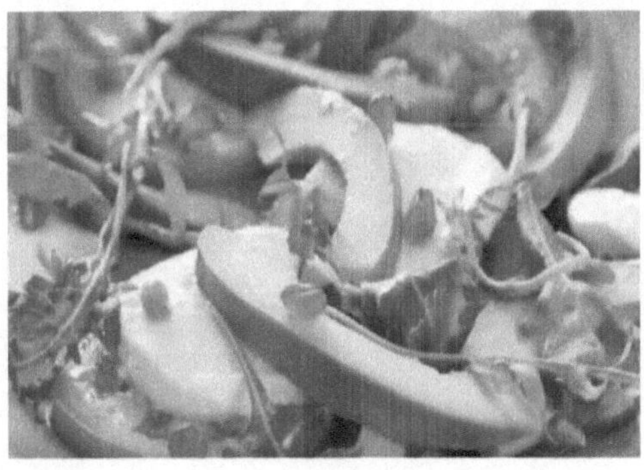

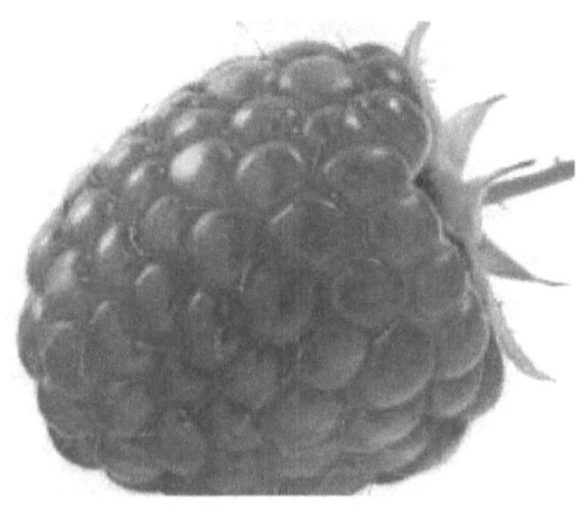

Training 10.00

Coconut water

Or mackerel paste with roasted peppers and olives

After workout

Cocktail with avocado banana and raw yolks and coconut water

Lunch

Tomatoes, zucchini, blanched spinach, beef steak

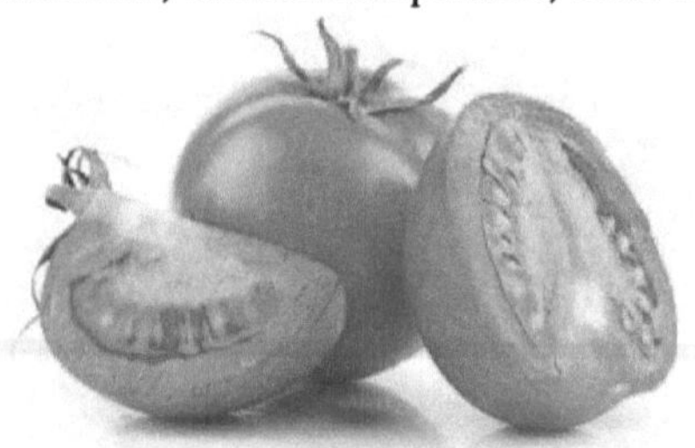

Tomatoes

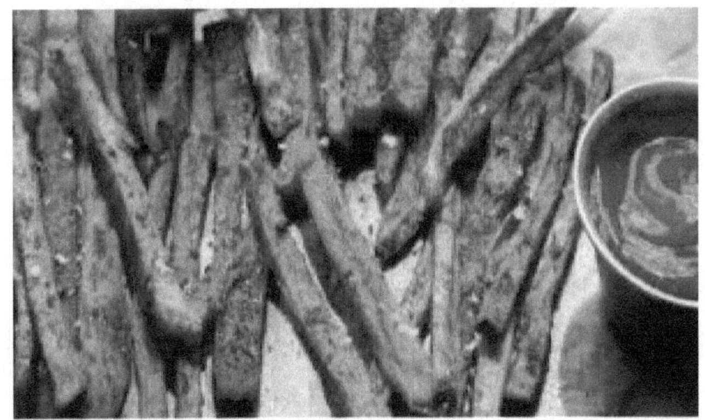

Zucchini

Dinner

Boiled vegetables (zucchini, broccoli, celery) with pork tenderloin stew in curry sauce on coconut milk and a leafy salad with a dressing made of balsamic vinegar
Tea, silage

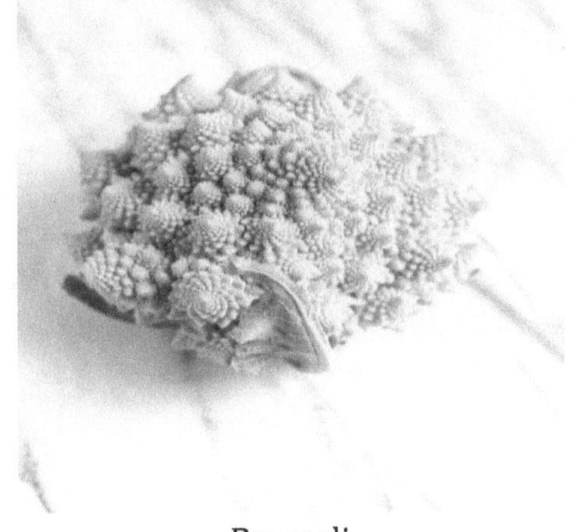

Broccoli

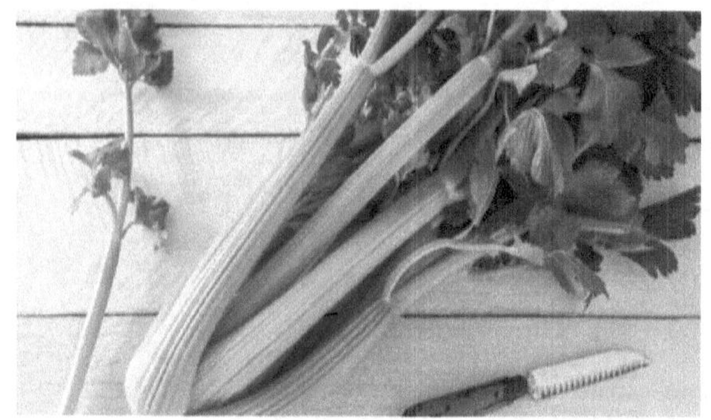

Celery

Supper

Steamed fish / baked in marinade with coconut milk, rosemary, sea salt, chilli

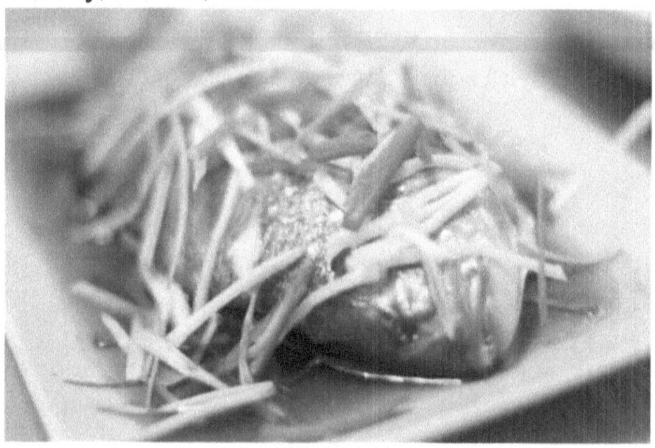

Steamed fish

CELEBRITIES ARE OBSESSED WITH THE KETOGENIC DIET

How celebrities like Meghan Markle, Gwyneth Paltrow, Ariana Grande, Kim Kardashian used Keto to transform their bodies and improve health

Meet 14 Celebrities Names Who Ditched Meat to Go Vegan or Vegetarian who are making us aspire to eat veg.

Meghan Markle

As rumour spread that Prince Harry has had his diet rebuild by Meghan Markle, however, is the Duchess of Sussex a vegetarian? When addressing Best Health in 2016 she expressed that when she was filming Suits, "I'm conscious of what I eat. I try to eat vegan during the week and after that have more flexibility with what I dive into at the ends of the week." So absolutely part time on the job, at that point!

Kim Kardashian

Kourtney's not by any means the only Kardashian who's been partaken in low-carb lifestyle. Kim has Joined the moving train, as well, and, as per report published in June 2016 in People, reportedly shed 60 pounds (lbs) after he gave birth to her child, Saint, while on the

Atkins 40 diet. Atkins 40 is a variant of the Atkins diet intended for individuals with under 40 lbs to lose, and has been around since the 1970s. Atkins is basically the first keto diet and involves a very limited intake of carbs and high amount of fat. The fundamental different is that on the Atkins diet you'll gradually reintroduce carbs, so ketosis likely will only come into play during stage 1.

Gwyneth Paltrow

Paltrow has been known to dole out pretty wacky wellbeing advice through her health lifestyle brand Goop, like recommending body stickers to ease anxiety, as People reported in August 2017. According to a 2017 Bravo story, the actress and business mogul is a fan of the keto diet, which has a lot more research backing it up than some of her other claims. An report on Goop stated what the diet is all about and how to determine whether it's the correct one for you.

Ariana Grande

The newly engaged songstress has been veggie lover since 2013. As stated in an interview published in December 2014 in The Mirror, she did the switch in light of her love for creatures. "I love animals more than I love most people, not kidding," she said. She's agreed that eating out can be muddled yet says her typical move is to order what she knows is vegetarian — veggies, fruit, plates of mixed greens — and afterward fill up on other things once she's home. She has also spoken out about animal rights, as PETA noted, and against using animal products, according to MindBodyGreen.

Jessica Chastain

After having low energy levels, the Golden Globe nominee went vegan. Telling W Magazine about the experience, Chastain stated, "I simply had more energy than I've ever had in my whole life. I was just listening to what my body was telling me!"

Liam Hemsworth

The youngest Hemsworth sibling, Miley Cyrus fiance, and The Hunger Games star reportedly went on vegan in 2015. The impetus? "My own wellbeing and after all the information gathered concerning the mistreatment of animals, I couldn't keep on eating meat," he said in an interview published in November 2015 in Men's Journal. "The more I knew about, the harder and harder it was to do.." He's stated that eating in this manner has helped him both physically and mentally, he's encouraged his oldest sibling, Chris Hemsworth, to try it out, as well.

Serena Williams

Popular player to ever get a tennis racquet, Serena Williams went on an extremely strict diet after having her baby girl, Alexis Olympia. Talking at a Wimbledon press conference, Serena stated, "I was veggie lover, I didn't eat sugar!" The result of her change in diet didn't yield the results until the point that she ceased bosom sustaining, remarking, " I shed 10 pounds in seven days when I stopped. I simply continued dropping."

Will.I.AM

The Black Eyed Peas hit maker, Will.I.AM went Vegan in early 2018, stating via his Instagram post that he had joined the 'V.gang' Catchy.

Vinny Guadagnino

Guadagnino returned into the spotlight in 2018 with the reboot of MTV's hit reality television show Jersey Shore, called Jersey Shore Family Reunion. In the six years since the MTV show last aired, PopSugar reported in May 2018 that Guadagnino has embraced the keto diet and Create an Instagram profile with @ketoguido. He suggests eating bacon, butter, steak, fatty fish, plants, and exercising every week. As indicated by March 8, 2018, Instagram post, Guadagnino says his old method for eating had him 50 lbs heavier and looking 10 years older.

Madonna

As report stated by The Cut, the sixty year old superstar follows a super strict vegan macrobiotic diet which consists of cold pressed juices, fruits, vegetables and whole grains like quinoa.

Lea Michele

Formal Glee star Lea Michele used to treats her body like a temple, and turned vegan for the health advantages and also animal rights reasons. "It's tied in being good to your body and the planet. I'm a foodie, however I believe it's much more fun to discover things on the menu that are beneficial for me," she said. Lea was respected by PETA in 2010 for her philanthropy work with animals.

Jared Leto

The Oscar-winning actor Jared Leto and the rest of his 30 Seconds To Mars bandmates are generally strict vegetarians. "Indeed, here was a time when we used to sacrifice goats, but then we all became vegans, so we've been sacrificing tofu before the shows!" Good to know, Jared.

Adriana Lima

It take nothing to get the body of a Victoria's Secret angel. A low-carb diet and two-hour workouts each day. That's apparently what Lima did to prep for the Victoria's Secret Fashion Show a few years back, In an article publish from The Cut. Her diet was primarily made up of green veggies, protein, and protein shakes or cereal bars as snacks. Since then, it seems she's stuck to a keto diet, according to a story published in September 2017 in Harper's Bazaar.

Paul McCartney

When the beloved Beatle posed for an ad for PETA in 2008, he stated the moment he turned vegetarian, ABC News reported: "Few years back, I was fishing, and as I was reeling in the poor fish, I realized, 'I am killing him — all for the passing pleasure it brings me.' And something inside me clicked. I realized as I watched him fight for breath that his life was as important to him as mine is to me."

THE 10 IMPORTANT THINGS YOU SHOULD KNOW ABOUT THE KETO LIFESTYLE BEFORE YOU START

Want to eat less sugar, lose weight, and change your metabolism? The ketogenic or keto diet might work for you.

Here are things you should know before going on keto.

Not All Fat Is 'Good' Fat

Put simply, following the keto diet involves eating mostly high-fat foods. But this doesn't mean you can eat more fast food and dessert. Foods like avocados, eggs, and nuts count as optimal fat sources on this diet. Butter, cream, and other high-fat dairy and meat products do not.

It isn't a high-protein diet

On average, experts say protein should make up about 20% of your daily calorie intake. Recommendations don't change on keto. Instead, you're supposed to dedicate 75% of your calories from fat, 20% from protein, and only 5% from carbohydrates.

You're allowed to drink alcohol

Most alcoholic drinks are a low-carb dieter's worst enemy. But that doesn't mean you have to give up drinking entirely if you're on a keto diet.

Dry wines and light beers fall into the low- or no-carb category — you can have them as long as you drink responsibly. You won't lose weight if you spend all your calories on booze.

You shouldn't fast on the keto diet right away

When you first start the keto diet, your body won't quite know what's happening. It's best to make sure you're eating enough to properly adjust to the upcoming metabolic shift before making any more major changes.

This doesn't mean you can't incorporate methods like intermittent fasting into your diet once your body adjusts to ketosis. Just don't rush into it.

You don't have to stop exercising on keto

Whether this is good news to you or not — yes, a diet that discourages exercise IS too good to be true — you shouldn't avoid creating a workout schedule. Working out on this diet can be completely safe, as long as you keep them short, don't exert yourself too much, and switch things up from day to day.

You'll probably lose weight — at first

One dietitian tried the keto diet herself after more

clients started asking about it. She said that even though effects like weight loss are certainly possible in the short-term, researchers aren't sure the same thing frequently happens in the long-term. Not many people stick with it that long.

Your gut may suffer

It's also difficult to include prebiotic foods such as onions, garlic, bananas and oats on a very low-carb, high-fat diet. "These foods encourage good growth of bacteria that support our intestinal health, which is tied to our overall health," says Julie Stefanski, a registered dietitian and spokesperson for the Academy of Nutrition and Dietetics. "But we don't know yet how the lack of fiber on a ketogenic diet impacts our microbiome or gastrointestinal health long-term."

You can't actually eat as much as you want

The keto diet forces you to cut back on many of the snack foods, desserts, and other high-carb options that could have made weight loss difficult for you in the past. But that doesn't mean you can eat infinite amounts of bacon and coconut oil. Consuming more calories, whether healthy or not, doesn't work.

Keto forces your body into a state of ketosis

When your body enters a state of ketosis, it burns fat as a primary energy source instead of carbohydrates.

That's why you have to eat more fat and fewer carbs to reach this point. Ketosis is different from ketoacidosis — a life-threatening condition some people with diabetes develop.

Keto isn't the best weight loss diet for everyone

When Kirkpatrick tried the keto diet, she too experienced flu-like symptoms, which isn't an uncommon side effect when going on such a drastic diet. Chances are, you'll feel fatigued, you'll crave sugar obsessively, and you'll get a little "hangry." Headaches and nausea are also possible downsides.

Some dieters can't make it past these hurdles, and go back to their former eating habits.

THE BIGGEST MISTAKE PEOPLE MAKE WHILE BEING ON VEGAN KETO

It can be frustrating reading how others are successful with keto and you can't seem to be making any form of progress.

Fortunately, it's usually just a small thing preventing you from achieving your goals.

Below are some of the most common mistakes made by people that are starting a keto diet.

Too Much Protein

In a keto diet, you are going to need more fat than protein. Sometimes it seems as though some people forget this. They try to consume just as much protein as fat.

Doing this is going to slow down the weight loss process if that is your ultimate goal.

Having enough protein is really important for all of your muscles to function properly. However, consuming too much protein will cause your body to start turning some of it into glucose. The last thing you want to do when you're trying to eliminate sugars from your body is to have it make sugar from too much protein.

When you eat the right amount of protein, you'll be able to hold onto some of that protein instead of it being converted into glucose. This means your muscles will have some protein to use when it needs to.

It's not meant to be a permanent way of eating.

Although many people find weight loss success on the ketogenic diet, it's not a way of eating that's meant to be permanent. Due to its many restrictions, it can be difficult to do normal day-to-day things like go to drinks with friends or have dinner with family.

"Think of it as something you're going to do anywhere from eight to 12, to maybe 16 weeks," Mancinelli said. And continue to maintain a healthy, well-balanced diet after that.

Comparing Yourself to Others

Sometimes it's difficult, especially with the age we live in, to not compare yourself to others. However, when you're dieting, comparing yourself to others is one of the last things you need to do.

This is similar to the scale mistake talked about earlier. When you compare yourself to others, you're more than likely going to start stressing about the diet and have trouble focusing on it.

Stress has a major effect on your body whether you're

dieting or not. You may not recognize how much it causes your body to change, but it makes a massive difference. If you're constantly stressed, you'll notice that your weight won't change as much as it probably should be.

On a keto diet, your body is going to react to it differently than the person next to you. That is why it is pointless to compare yourself to somebody else dieting. Everybody's body is different and will change different on any diet.

Focus on yourself when you're on a keto diet. If you aren't losing the weight right away, don't panic. The change is coming shortly. Keep your mind off the scale and stick with the diet and you won't be able to recognize yourself in a few short weeks.

Going About It By Yourself

Any diet is hard, but going about it by yourself will make the journey that much more difficult. Almost everything is easier when you have somebody to share it with.

When you have those moments of weakness (trust me, you'll have them no matter what) it'll be nice to have somebody there with you to keep you strong. If you and somebody else are embarking on the same journey, staying accountable for everything you do becomes easier.

Trying to hold yourself accountable can become difficult at times. When you have another person close to you to hold you accountable, staying with the diet becomes more of a goal instead of a daunting task which is always a plus.

Having somebody else with you on this journey allows you to share all of your struggles and successes with a person going through the same thing as you.

Not Enough Fats

When you start a keto diet, you will be consuming plenty of fats. However, there are many instances where not enough fats are consumed.

Growing up on a diet that was relatively low in fat and switching to a diet that is supposed to be high in fat could take some getting used to. You might feel as though you are eating too many fats, but more than likely, you're not.

This is why it is important to track your meals and see if you're meeting your daily macro goals.

It's important to just trust the process of the keto diet. Follow your macros even if it feels like you're eating more than you should.

You have your macros for a reason and sticking to that will give you the best chance at reaching your goals in a suitable time frame.

Looking For a Quick Fix

Some people think that going on a keto diet and cutting carbs is going to solve all of their weight problems fast and they can go back to their old lifestyles when it comes to food. This is false.

Starting a keto diet is something that you really shouldn't use if you want a quick solution to your weight problems. Yes, you'll lose weight in the first few weeks, but if you go back to your old habits, the weight will come back in a hurry.

Ketogenic diets are lifestyle changes, not just changes for a few weeks. Switch to a different diet if you want to lose weight quickly without changing your eating habits too much. Don't waste your time and money on a keto diet when it's going to last weeks and not years.

HOW TO LOSE 30LBS IN FEW WEEKS WITHOUT DOING HARMFUL EXERCISES

It is possible to lose 30 lbs. of bodyfat in few weeks by optimizing any of three factors: diet, or drug/supplement regimen. In this book, we'll explore ways to lose bodyfat without exercise.

Avoid "White" Carbohydrates

Avoid any carbohydrate that is — or can be — white. The following foods are thus prohibited, except for within 1.5 hours of finishing a resistance-training workout of at least 20 minutes in length: bread, rice, cereal, potatoes, pasta, and fried food with breading. If you avoid eating anything white, you'll be safe.

Eat The Same Few Meals Over And Over Again

The most successful dieters, regardless of whether their goal is muscle gain or fat loss, eat the same few meals over and over again. Mix and match, constructing each meal with one from each of the three following groups:

Proteins:

- Chicken breast or thigh
- Grass-fed organic beef
- Pork

Legumes:

- Lentils
- Black beans
- Pinto beans

Vegetables:

- Spinach
- Asparagus
- Peas

Mixed vegetables

Eat as much as you like of the above food items. Just remember: keep it simple. Pick three or four meals and repeat them. Almost all restaurants can give you a salad or vegetables in place of french fries or potatoes. Surprisingly, I have found Mexican food, swapping out rice for vegetables, to be one of the cuisines most conducive to the "slow carb" diet.

Most people who go on "low" carbohydrate diets complain of low energy and quit, not because such diets can't work, but because they consume insufficient calories. A 1/2 cup of rice is 300 calories, whereas a 1/2 cup of spinach is 15 calories! Vegetables are not calorically dense, so it is critical that you add legumes for caloric load.

Some athletes eat 6-8x per day to break up caloric load and avoid fat gain. I think this is ridiculously inconvenient. I eat 4x per day:

- 10 am – breakfast
- 1pm – lunch
- 5pm – smaller second lunch
- 7:30-9pm – sports training
- 10pm – dinner
- 12am – glass of wine and Discovery Channel before bed

Here are some of my meals that recur again and again:

Breakfast

Scrambled Eggology pourable egg whites with one whole egg, black beans, and microwaved mixed vegetables

Lunch

Grass-fed organic beef, pinto beans, mixed vegetables, and extra guacamole (Mexican restaurant)

Dinner

Grass-fed organic beef (from Trader Joe's), lentils, and mixed vegetables

Don't Drink Calories

Drink massive quantities of water and as much unsweetened iced tea, tea, diet sodas, coffee (without white cream), or other no-calorie/low-calorie beverages as you like. Do not drink milk, normal soft drinks, or fruit juice.

Take One Day Off Per Week

I recommend Saturdays as your "Dieters Gone Wild" day. Paradoxically, dramatically spiking caloric intake in this way once per week increases fat loss by ensuring that your metabolic rate (thyroid function, etc.) doesn't downregulate from extended caloric restriction. That's right: eating pure crap can help you lose fat.

A LIST OF KETO-FRIENDLY AND TASTY KETO-FRIENDLY RECIPES

Vegan recipes are like gold. Especially when they feature whole foods, and lots of plants. This type of cooking benefit your health and overall well-being in many important ways. No meat? No dairy? Don't sweat it. There are many other ingredients to get excited about when you're cooking and eating.

Here are some Keto Vegan Recipe you can start cooking in your home.

BREAKFAST

Keto Fat Bombs

These fat bombs are your best friend. Don't let the name scare you—these little balls are the perfect way to curb your hunger.

Yields: 8
Prep Time: 0 hours 5 mins
Total Time: 0 hours 25 mins

Ingredients

- 8 oz. cream cheese, softened to room temperature
- 1/2 c. keto-friendly peanut butter
- 1/4 c. coconut oil, plus 2 tbsp.
- 1/2 tsp. kosher salt
- 1 c. keto-friendly dark chocolate chips (such as Lily's)

Instructions

- Line a small baking sheet with parchment paper. In a medium bowl, combine cream cheese, peanut butter, ¼ c coconut oil, and salt. Using a hand mixer, beat mixture until fully combined, about 2 minutes. Place bowl in freezer to firm up slightly, 10 to 15 minutes.

- When peanut butter mixture has hardened, use a small cookie scoop or spoon to create golf ball sized balls. Place in the refrigerator to harden, 5 minutes.
- Meanwhile, make chocolate drizzle: combine chocolate chips and remaining coconut oil in a microwave safe bowl and microwave in 30-second intervals until fully melted. Drizzle over peanut butter balls and place back in the refrigerator to harden, 5 minutes. Serve.
- To store, keep covered in refrigerator.

Nutrition Info

Per Serving: 84 calories; 8.4 g fat; 2.6 g carbohydrates; 2 g protein; 0 mg cholesterol; 0 mg sodium

Chocolate-Raspberry Chia Pudding Shots

Dessert and breakfast, together once more! These Chocolate-Raspberry Chia pudding shots are relatively similar to enchantment. They're solid and sweet - the ideal mix. Celebrated for being a low carb thickening agent, these natural chia seeds make a remarkable pudding!

Prep Time 1 hour;
Servings 2; Calories 240 kcal

Ingredients:

- ¼ cup chia seeds
- 1/2 cup coconut milk
- 1/4 cup almond milk
- 1 tablespoon cacao powder
- 1 tablespoon Stevia
- 1/2 cup raspberries

Instructions:

1. In a container, bring together all the ingredients (with the exception of the raspberries) and shake vivaciously. Let sit for 2 minutes and after that fill four shot glasses.

2. Refrigerate for no less than 60 minutes (ideally across the night) until the point that blend thickens into pudding. Top with raspberries.

Recipe Notes:

This yield of this recipe is 4 shots. 1 serving is 2 shots.

Nutritional Information:

Calories: 241, Protein: 4g Fats: 20g, Net Carbs

Curry Tofu Scramble With Avocado

This tofu scramble is a fabulous low carb veggie lover approach to begin the morning, with a lot of supplements and sufficient calories to give you vitality for the day ahead.

Prep Time 5 minutes;
Total Time 20 minutes, Cook Time 13 minutes; Calories 380 kcal Servings 3

Ingredients:

- 1 tbsp coconut oil
- 2 tbsp olive oil
- 300 g tofu (extra firm)
- 1 tsp turmeric
- 1 tbsp nutritional yeast
- 1 tbsp curry powder
- 1/2 cup zucchini (chopped)
- 1 cup mushrooms (chopped)
- 1 tomato (chopped)
- cilantro (optional)(to garnish)
- 300-gram avocado

Instructions:

- The initial step is to dry the tofu so it ingests the flavor.
- Cut the tofu into 1 inch long strips, spread out the strips on a paper towel,

- put another paper towel to finish everything and after that a slashing board.
- Place something substantial over this, for example, a few books.
- Abandon it to sit for around 15 minutes.
- Add the coconut oil to the dish and disintegrate the tofu into the skillet with your hands.
- Cook for around 5 minutes, mixing every now and again.
- Include the turmeric, nourishing yeast and curry powder and 1 tbsp of the olive oil,
- blend and cook for a further 4 minutes.
- Add whatever remains of the olive oil, zucchini, mushroom and tomato and sear for a further 4 minutes blending much of the time.
- Serve with 1 little medium size avocado (roughly 100g) cut.

Recipe Notes:

This meal can be refrigerated for a few days.

Nutritional Information:
Calories: 381, Fats: 32g, Protein: 11g, Net Carbs:

Curry Tofu Scramble with Avocado

This tofu scramble is a fabulous low carb veggie lover approach to begin the morning, with a lot of supplements and sufficient calories togive you vitality for the day ahead.

Prep Time 5 minutes;
Cook Time 13 minutes;
Total Time 20 minutes,
Calories 380 kcal
Servings 3

Ingredients:

- 1 tbsp coconut oil
- 2 tbsp olive oil
- 300 g tofu (extra firm)
- 1 tsp turmeric
- 1 tbsp nutritional yeast
- 1 tbsp curry powder
- 1/2 cup zucchini (chopped)
- 1 cup mushrooms (chopped)
- 1 tomato (chopped)
- cilantro (optional)(to garnish)
- 300-gram avocado

Instructions

- The initial step is to dry the tofu so it ingests the flavor.

- Cut the tofu into 1 inch long strips, spread out the strips on a paper towel,
- put another paper towel to finish everything and after that a slashing board.
- Place something substantial over this, for example, a few books.
- Abandon it to sit for around 15 minutes.
- Add the coconut oil to the dish and disintegrate the tofu into the skillet with your hands.
- Cook for around 5 minutes, mixing every now and again.
- Include the turmeric, nourishing yeast and curry powder and 1 tbsp of the olive oil,
- blend and cook for a further 4 minutes.
- Add whatever remains of the olive oil, zucchini, mushroom and tomato and sear for a further 4 minutes blending much of the time.
- Serve with 1 little medium size avocado (roughly 100g) cut.

Recipe Notes:
This meal can be refrigerated for a few days.
Nutritional Information:
Calories: 381, Fats: 32g, Protein: 11g, Net Carbs: 8g

Chocolate-Raspberry Chia Pudding Shots

Dessert and breakfast, together once more! These Chocolate-Raspberry Chia pudding shots are relatively similar to enchantment. They're solid and sweet - the ideal mix. Celebrated for being a low carb thickening agent, these natural chia seeds make a remarkable pudding!

Prep Time 1 hour;
Servings 2; Calories 240 kcal

Ingredients:

- ¼ cup chia seeds
- 1/2 cup coconut milk
- 1/4 cup almond milk
- 1 tablespoon cacao powder
- 1 tablespoon Stevia
- 1/2 cup raspberries

Instructions:

- In a container, bring together all the ingredients (with the exception of the raspberries) and shake vivaciously. Let sit for 2 minutes and after that fill four shot glasses.

- Refrigerate for no less than 60 minutes (ideally across the night) until the point that blend thickens into pudding. Top with raspberries.

Recipe Notes:

This yield of this recipe is 4 shots. 1 serving is 2 shots.

Nutritional Information:
Calories: 241, Protein: 4g Fats: 20g, , Net Carbs: 4g

Blackberry Coconut Breakfast Bowl

This breakfast bowl is smooth and rich, and has the magnificent FLAVORS of blackberry and coconut. An extraordinary begin to the day. It's likewise super simple and snappy to get ready!

Total Time 5 minutes;
Prep Time 5 minutes;
Calories 467 kcal;
Servings 2

Ingredients:

- 1 cup blackberries
- 1 cup coconut milk
- 3 tbsp ground flaxseed
- 1/4 cup water
- 1 cup spinach
- 1/4 cup coconut flakes
- 2 tbsp chia seeds

Instructions:

1. Mix the flaxseed with the water in a glass until the point that the water is assimilated (just needs around 10 seconds).
2. Pour a large portion of the blackberries (sparing some for trimming), coconut drain, spinach and the flaxseed blend into a blender and mix until smooth.

3. In a different sear the coconut drops for a moment or two on high warmth to toast them.
4. Pour the berry blend into two dishes and sprinkle the rest of the ground flaxseed on top alongside the chia seeds and coconut pieces. Appreciate promptly.

Recipe Notes:
You can store the blackberry blend in the ice chest and utilize it the following day in the event that you like. Note this formula makes two servings - the beneath dietary data is for one serving.

Nutritional Information:

Calories: 465, Fats: 43g, Protein: 8g, Net Carbs: 7g

LUNCH

Keto Chicken Enchilada Bowl

This Keto Chicken Enchilada Bowl is a low carb twist on a Mexican favorite!

Prep Time: 20 minutes
Cook Time: 30 minutes
Total Time: 50 minutes
Yield: 4 servings

Ingredients

- 2 tablespoons coconut oil (for searing chicken)
- 1 pound of boneless, skinless chicken thighs
- 3/4 cup red enchilada sauce (recipe from Low Carb Maven)
- 1/4 cup water
- 1/4 cup chopped onion
- 4 oz can diced green chiles

Toppings (feel free to customize)

- 1 whole avocado, diced
- 1 cup shredded cheese (I used mild cheddar)
- 1/4 cup chopped pickled jalapenos
- 1/2 cup sour cream
- 1 roma tomato, chopped

Optional: serve over plain cauliflower rice (or Mexican cauliflower rice) for a more complete meal!

Instructions

- In a pot or dutch oven over medium heat melt the coconut oil. Once hot, sear chicken thighs until lightly brown.

- Pour in enchilada sauce and water then add onion and green chiles. Reduce heat to a simmer and cover. Cook chicken for 17-25 minutes or until chicken is tender and fully cooked through to at least 165 degrees internal temperature.

- Carefully remove the chicken and place onto a work surface. Chop or shred chicken (your preference) then add it back into the pot. Let the chicken simmer uncovered for an additional 10 minutes to absorb flavor and allow the sauce to reduce a little.

- To Serve, top with avocado, cheese, jalapeno, sour cream, tomato, and any other desired toppings. Feel free to customize these to your preference. Serve alone or over cauliflower rice if desired just be sure to update your personal nutrition info as needed.

Nutrition Info

Calories: 568 Calories

Total Carbs: 10.41g

Fiber: 4.27g

Net Carbs: 6.14g

Protein: 38.38g

Fat: 40.21g

Almond Coconut Curry on Veges

This almond coconut curry is super speedy and simple and tastes extraordinary as well! It flaunts nutritious vegetables alongside solid fats and a decent calorie tally.

Time 15 minutes; Total Time 15 minutes;
Servings 4; Calories 439 kcal

Ingredients:

For the veges
For the curry

- 1 tsp coconut oil
- 400 ml coconut milk
- 2 cups mushrooms
- 125 g almond butter (100% ground almonds)
- 4 cups spinach
- 1 tbsp tomato paste
- 2 cups brocolli (chopped into florets)
- 1 tbsp curry powder

Instructions:

For the curry mixture

- Put the coconut drain, almond spread, tomato glue and curry powder in a blender. Mix for around 20 seconds or until smooth.

- Add the curry blend to a pan on low-medium warmth and warmth for 10-15 minutes or until warmed through. Blend habitually to abstain from staying.

For the veges

- Heat the coconut oil in a container on medium-high warmth and include the broccoli and mushrooms. Sear for around 3 minutes. Include the spinach and warmth for one more moment.

- Serve the veges in a bowl with the curry blend poured over the best.

Recipe Notes:

You can make the almond margarine by granulating almonds in a sustenance processor.

The curry blend isolates whenever left to sit in the refrigerator for some time, so make certain to mix it completely before utilizing on the off chance that you have put away it in the ice chest.

Nutritional Information:
Calories: 438, Fats: 41g, Protein: 11g, Net Carbs: 9g

Sesame Salmon w. Baby Bok Choy & Mushrooms

Ingredients

Main Dish

- 4 each 4-6 oz. salmon fillet
- 2 each portobello mushroom caps (or 8 oz. baby bella mushrooms)
- 4 each baby bok choy
- 1 tbsp toasted sesame seeds
- 1 ea green onion

Marinade

- 1 tbsp olive oil
- 1 tsp sesame oil
- 1 tbsp Coconut Aminos
- 1/2 inch Ginger grated (approx. 1 tsp.)
- 1/2 lemon juice
- 1/2 tsp Salt
- 1/2 tsp black pepper

Instructions

- Whisk together all of your marinade ingredients
- Drizzle half of the marinade on the salmon and turn to coat. Cover and refrigerate the salmon

while it marinates for one hour.

- Preheat oven to 400.
- Prepare vegetables: Trim the rough ends from the bok choy and cut into halves. Slice the mushrooms into ½ inch pieces.
- Drizzle the remaining marinade over the vegetables and lay on a lined baking sheet.
- Place salmon, skin side down, on a lined baking sheet as well. Bake until salmon is cooked through, about 20 minutes.
- Top with sliced green onions and sesame seeds.

Caprese Tuna Salad Stuffed Tomatoes

Prep Time: 10 minutes
Yield: Serves 1
Serving Size: entire recipe
Calories per serving: 196
Fat per serving: 4.9g

Ingredients

- 1 medium tomato
- 1 (5oz) can tuna, very well drained
- 2 tsp balsamic vinegar
- 1 TBSP chopped mozzarella {1/4 oz.}
- 1 TBSP chopped fresh basil
- 1 TBSP chopped green onion

Instructions

- Cut the top 1/4-inch off the tomato. Use a spoon to scoop out the insides of the tomato. Set aside while you make the tuna salad.
- Stir together the drained tuna, balsamic vinegar, mozzarella, basil, and green onion. Put the tuna salad in the hollowed out tomato, and enjoy!
- Note: I prefer using fresh mozzarella but any mozzarella is good in here.

Loaded Chicken Salad

A delicious salad filled with plenty of vegetables and delicious grilled meat!

Prep Time 10 minutes
Cook Time 8 minutes
Total Time 18 minutes
Total Carbs 12.86g

Ingredients

- 1 boneless chicken breast (about 300g, with or without skin)
- 1 tbsp extra virgin olive oil
- 1/4 tsp Himalayan salt
- 1/4 tsp black pepper
- 1 avocado
- 100 g mozzarella balls
- 1 large tomato (any colour)
- 1 har artichoke hearts (my jar was 170g)
- 1/2 red onion
- 5 asparagus
- 20 leaves basil
- 4 cups baby spinach (200g used)

Dressing

- 2 tbsp extra virgin olive oil
- 1 1/2 tbsp balsamic vinegar

- 1 tsp dijon mustard
- 1 clove garlic
- pinch Himalayan salt
- pinch black pepper

Instructions

- Peel and dice the avocado. Slice the red onion. Dice the tomato. Pile the basil leaves together, roll them up and slice. Cut the stems off the asparagus and slice in half. Mince the garlic.
- Slice the chicken breast in half lengthwise. Sprinkle the 1/4 tsp of salt and pepper on each sides. Heat the 1 tbsp of olive oil in a cast iron skillet and place the chicken breasts in. Fry on each side, about 3 minutes each side, until they have a nice golden brown colour and cooked through. Add the asparagus beside the chicken breasts and cook a few minutes until soft and grilled. Take out the chicken and slice.
- In a small bowl, combine the minced garlic, olive oil, balsamic vinegar, dijon, and salt & pepper.
- Add the baby spinach to a large bowl or plate. Cover with the grilled chicken, avocado, mozzarella, tomatoes, artichoke, red onions, asparagus and basil leaves. Pour the dressing over and enjoy!

Notes

You can add 1 tbsp of honey to the salad dressing if you don't mind the extra carbs or want a sweeter dressing.

Nutrition Info
Calories 430 Calories from Fat 264
Saturated Fat 6.57g 33%
Total Carbohydrates 12.86g 4%
Dietary Fiber 6.12g 24%
Sugars 3.16g

DINNER

Keto Instant Pot Crack Chicken Recipe

Rich, creamy, and full of flavor, this Keto Instant Pot Crack Chicken Recipe is sure to be a favorite family dinner.

Cuisine: American
Prep time: 5 mins
Cook time: 20 mins
Total time: 25 mins
Serves: 8 servings (yields about 7 cups total)

Ingredients

- 2 slices bacon, chopped
- 2 lbs (910 g) boneless, skinless chicken breasts
- 2 (8 oz/227 g) blocks cream cheese
- ½ cup (120 ml) water
- 2 tablespoons apple cider vinegar
- 1 tablespoon dried chives
- 1½ teaspoons garlic powder
- 1½ teaspoons onion powder
- 1 teaspoon crushed red pepper flakes
- 1 teaspoon dried dill
- ¼ teaspoon salt
- ¼ teaspoon black pepper
- ½ cup (2 oz/57 g) shredded cheddar
- 1 scallion, green and white parts, thinly sliced

Instructions

- Turn pressure cooker on, press "Sauté", and wait 2 minutes for the pot to heat up. Add the chopped bacon and cook until crispy. Transfer to a plate and set aside. Press "Cancel" to stop sautéing.
- Add the chicken, cream cheese, water, vinegar, chives, garlic powder, onion powder, crushed red pepper flakes, dill, salt, and black pepper to the pot. Turn the pot on Manual, High Pressure for 15 minutes and then do a quick release.
- Use tongs to transfer the chicken to a large plate, shred it with 2 forks, and return it back to the pot.
- Stir in the cheddar cheese.
- Top with the crispy bacon and scallion, and serve.

Notes

We've tested this recipe upwards of 10 times and have never had the burn warning come on; however, several readers have had the warning come on, so we want to give a tip. In step 1 of the Instructions above, after removing the bacon from the pot, we recommend adding a splash of water, and use a wooden spoon to scrape up any brown bits that have formed on the bottom to deglaze the pan. After that, continue on with step 1 and press "Cancel" to stop sauteing.

Nutrition Facts

Calories: 437 Fat: 27.6 Potassium: 390 Net Carbs: 4.3 Carbohydrates: 4.5 Sodium: 420 Fiber: .2 Protein: 41.2

Keto Chicken Enchilada Bowl

This Keto Chicken Enchilada Bowl is a low carb twist on a Mexican favorite! It's So easy to make, totally filling and ridiculously yummy!

Prep Time: 20 minutes
Cook Time: 30 minutes
Total Time: 50 minutes
Yield: 4 servings

Ingredients

- 2 tablespoons coconut oil (for searing chicken)
- 1 pound of boneless, skinless chicken thighs
- 3/4 cup red enchilada sauce (recipe from Low Carb Maven)
- 1/4 cup water
- 1/4 cup chopped onion
- 4 oz can diced green chiles

Toppings (feel free to customize)

- 1 whole avocado, diced
- 1 cup shredded cheese (I used mild cheddar)
- 1/4 cup chopped pickled jalapenos
- 1/2 cup sour cream
- 1 roma tomato, chopped

Optional: serve over plain cauliflower rice (or mexican cauliflower rice) for a more complete meal!

Instructions

- In a pot or dutch oven over medium heat melt the coconut oil. Once hot, sear chicken thighs until lightly brown.

- Pour in enchilada sauce and water then add onion and green chiles. Reduce heat to a simmer and cover. Cook chicken for 17-25 minutes or until chicken is tender and fully cooked through to at least 165 degrees internal temperature.

- Careully remove the chicken and place onto a work surface. Chop or shred chicken (your preference) then add it back into the pot. Let the chicken simmer uncovered for an additional 10 minutes to absorb flavor and allow the sauce to reduce a little.

- To Serve, top with avocado, cheese, jalapeno, sour cream, tomato, and any other desired toppings. Feel free to customize these to your preference. Serve alone or over cauliflower rice if desired just be sure to update your personal nutrition info as needed.

Nutrition Info

Calories: 568 Calories
Total Carbs: 10.41g
Fiber: 4.27g
Net Carbs: 6.14g
Protein: 38.38g
Fat: 40.21g

Crab Stuffed Mushrooms With Cream Cheese

An easy recipe for crab stuffed mushrooms with cream cheese. Low carb, keto, and gluten free.

Prep Time 15 minutes
Cook Time 30 minutes
Servings 4 servings
Calories 160 kcal

Ingredients

- 20 ounces cremini (baby bella) mushrooms (20-25 individual mushrooms)
- 2 tablespoons finely grated parmesan cheese
- 1 tablespoon chopped fresh parsley
- salt

Filling:

- 4 ounces cream cheese softened to room temperature
- 4 ounces crab meat finely chopped
- 5 cloves garlic minced
- 1 teaspoon dried oregano
- 1/2 teaspoon paprika
- 1/2 teaspoon black pepper
- 1/4 teaspoon salt

Instructions

- Preheat the oven to 400 F. Prepare a baking sheet lined with parchment paper.
- Snap stems from mushrooms, discarding the stems and placing the mushroom caps on the baking sheet 1 inch apart from each other. Season the mushroom caps with salt.
- In a large mixing bowl, combine all filling ingredients and stir until well-mixed without any lumps of cream cheese. Stuff the mushroom caps with the mixture. Evenly sprinkle parmesan cheese on top of the stuffed mushrooms.
- Bake at 400 F until the mushrooms are very tender and the stuffing is nicely browned on top, about 30 minutes. Top with parsley and serve while hot.

Nutrition Notes

This recipe yields 5 g net carbs per serving (5-6 stuffed mushrooms).

Nutrition Info
Calories 160
Total Carb 5.5g 2%
Dietary Fiber 0.5g 1%
Sugars 0g
Protein 9g

Blueberry Fat Bombs

Makes 12 fat bombs / Prep time: 10 minutes, plus 3 hours chilling time

The shade of these fat bombs is a particular blue, which you may discover startling in light of the fact that not very many nourishments are blue. Frozen unsweetened berries will work if fresh are not available or in season: Just thaw the frozen fruit first. On the off chance that your zone has wild blueberries, use these little berries since they have an altogether more elevated amount of antioxidants against free radicals than grown blueberries.

Ingredients

- ½ cup coconut oil, at room temperature
- ½ cup cream cheese, at room temperature
- ½ cup blueberries, mashed with a fork
- 6 drops liquid stevia

Pinch ground nutmeg

Instructions

- Line a smaller scale biscuit tin with paper liners and put aside.
- In a medium bowl, stir together the coconut oil

and cream cheese until well blended.

- Stir in the blueberries, stevia, and nutmeg until combined.
- Divide the blueberry mixture into the muffin cups and place the tray in the freezer until set, about 3 hours.
- Place the fat bombs in an airtight container and store in the freezer until you wish to eat them.

Spiced-Chocolate Fat Bombs

Makes 12 fat bombs / Prep time: 10 minutes, plus 15 minutes chilling time / Cook time: 4 minutes

Great quality cocoa powder is an adequate ingredient on the keto-vegan diet, which implies you can, in any case, appreciate a chocolate pastry and bite when you require a fix. Dull chocolate, for example, cocoa is high in manganese, magnesium, copper, iron, and fiber and also cancer prevention agents, which battle free radicals in the body. Dim chocolate has been found to enable lower to circulatory strain, diminish cholesterol, and enhance intellectual capacity.

Ingredients

- ¾ **cup coconut oil**
- ¼ **cup cocoa powder**
- ¼ **cup almond butter**
- ⅛ **teaspoon chili powder**
- **3 drops liquid stevia**

Instructions

- Line a small scale biscuit tin with paper liners and put aside.

- Put a little pan over low warmth and include the coconut oil, cocoa powder, almond spread, stew powder, and stevia. Warmth until the point when the coconut oil is dissolved, at that point race to mix.

- Spoon the blend into the biscuit containers and place the tin in the fridge until the point when the bombs are firm around 15 minutes.

- Exchange the glasses to a hermetically sealed holder and store the fat bombs in the cooler until the point when you need to serve them.

Chocolate-Coconut Treats

Makes 16 treats / Prep time: 10 minutes, plus 30 minutes chilling time / Cook time: 3 minutes

Chocolate and coconut is a flawless combination often found in candy bars and many desserts. If you want a more elegant presentation, omit the coconut in step 3 and roll the semi-hardened chocolate mixture into balls instead of spreading it in a pan. Then roll the balls in the shredded coconut and place the treats in the freezer to firm up completely.

Ingredients

- ⅓ cup coconut oil
- ¼ cup unsweetened cocoa powder
- 4 drops liquid stevia Pinch sea salt
- ¼ cup shredded unsweetened coconut

Instructions

- Line a 6-by-6-inch baking dish with parchment paper and set aside.

- In a small saucepan over low heat, stir together the coconut oil, cocoa, stevia, and salt for about 3 minutes.
- Stir in the coconut and press the mixture into the baking dish.
- Place the baking dish in the refrigerator until

the mixture is hard, about 30 minutes.

- Cut into 16 pieces and store the treats in an airtight container in a cool place.

PREP TIP For a more finished look, you can spoon the hot mixture into candy molds instead of a baking dish. Pop the molds in the refrigerator for 30 minutes or until firm and pop the treats out into a cont

Almond Butter Fudge

Makes 36 pieces / Prep time: 10 minutes, plus 2 hours chilling time

Fudge ought to be smooth and thick with no coarseness or graininess. Since you won't utilize granulated sugar for this treat, the odds of misunderstanding the surface are incredibly diminished. Almond spread is an excellent wellspring of protein, nutrient E, iron, manganese, and fiber. On the off chance that you are not a devotee of this nut margarine, nutty spread or cashew margarine would likewise be flavorful and make the equivalent enticing outcomes.

Ingredients

- 1 cup coconut oil, at room temperature
- 1 cup almond butter
- ¼ Cup heavy cream
- ¼ Pinch sea salt
- 10 Drops liquid stevia

Instructions

- Line a 6-by-6-inch baking dish with parchment paper and set aside.

- In a medium bowl, whisk together the coconut oil, almond butter, heavy cream, stevia, and salt until very smooth.

- Spoon the mixture into the baking dish and smooth the top with a spatula.
- Place the dish in the refrigerator until the fudge is firm, about 2 hours.
- Cut into 36 pieces and store the fudge in an airtight container in the freezer for up to 2 weeks.

Peanut Butter Mousse

Serves 4 / Prep time: 10 minutes, plus 30 minutes chilling time

Peanut spread is dependably a convenient, delectable sandwich spread, however, it is utilized in numerous kinds of dishes everywhere throughout the world, and is extremely sound. Eating nutty spread, even in this delectable sweet, can decrease your danger of malignancy and coronary illness, and help bring down cholesterol levels. Common nutty spread is high in unsaturated fats, protein, fiber, and folate.

Ingredients

- 1 cup heavy (whipping) cream
- ¼ cup natural peanut butter
- 1 teaspoon alcohol-free pure vanilla extract
- 4 drops liquid stevia

Instructions

- In a medium bowl, beat together the heavy cream, peanut butter, vanilla, and stevia until firm peaks form, about 5 minutes.

- Spoon the mousse into 4 bowls and place in the refrigerator to chill for 30 minutes.

- Serve.

OTHER KETO VEGAN RECIPE

Cauliflower Pizza Crust

Prep Time 10 minutes
Cook Time 1 hour 10 minutes
Total Time 1 hour 20 minutes
Servings 6 1/2 " crusts
Calories 340 kcal

Ingredients

- 6 cups cauliflower florets 1 head
- 1 cup ground flax seeds
- 2 teaspoons basil
- 2 teaspoons oregano
- 1/2 cup nutritional yeast
- 2 tablespoons olive oil + more for oiling baking sheet
- 1 teaspoon onion powder
- 1 teaspoon garlic powder
- salt and pepper

Instructions

- Preheat oven to 400°.
- Steam cauliflower 10-15 minutes until tender. Let cool.
- In a cheesecloth or towel, squeeze out as much water as you can*. This will shrink the amount

of cauliflower to about 3 cups.

- Put cauliflower and the rest of ingredients into a food processor and mix thoroughly.
- Spread 1/4 of ingredients (depending upon the size of your pizza) onto an oiled baking sheet or parchment paper. With slightly wet hands (dough is sticky), spread out the dough to about 1/4" thick, pressing the cauliflower in firmly.
- Cook at 400° for 10 minutes. Flip over and cook another 10 minutes*.
- Add your toppings and cook for a few minutes, or store in the fridge and use within a few days!

Recipe Notes

If you prefer a flatbread texture that is not as crispy, don't squeeze out all the water. This way you will also get about twice as many crusts.

You may want to decrease the cooking time of the crust depending upon what toppings you are putting on it. My toppings didn't need much cooking time, so after the 20 minutes of cooking the crust, I only needed to cook my pizza for a few minutes to warm it up.

Nutrition Facts
Calories 340 Calories from Fat 216
Total Fat 24g 37%
Saturated Fat 2g 10%
Cholesterol 0mg 0%
Sugars 3g
Protein 13g 26%

Vegan Zucchini Lasagna with Tofu Ricotta and Walnut Sauce

Prep Time 10 minutes
Cook Time 35 minutes
Total Time 45 minutes
Servings 4
Calories 356 kcal

Ingredients

Walnut Sauce

- cup walnuts finely ground
- 1 25 ounce jar marinara sauce, divided
- 1/4 cup sun-dried tomatoes chopped

Lasagna

- Tofu Ricotta the whole batch
- zucchini
- tablespoons nutritional yeast optional

Instructions

- Preheat oven to 375°.
- Mix walnuts, marinara sauce (reserve 3/4 cup for the pan), and sun-dried tomatoes.
- Slice zucchini 1/16" lenthwise on a mandoline.
- In an 8x9" pan, pour 3/4 cup marinara sauce. Next, place zucchini noodles on marinara sauce,

overlapping each slice. Spread 1/3 of tofu ricotta over zucchini noodles. Sprinkle nutritional yeast on top of tofu ricotta. Pour 1/2 of walnut sauce on top.

- Layer more zucchini noodles, then 1/3 of tofu ricotta, nutritional yeast, and rest of walnut sauce. Finish with layer of zucchini noodles, tofu ricotta, and nutritional yeast. Bake at 375° for 35 minutes.

Nutrition Facts
Calories 356 Calories from Fat 225
Total Fat 25g 38%
Saturated Fat 1g 5%
Cholesterol 0mg 0%
Sugars 5g

Baked Tofu Fries

Prep Time 30 minutes
Cook Time 40 minutes
Total Time 1 hour 10 minutes
Servings people
Calories 132 kcal

Ingredients

- 15.5 ounces extra firm tofu drained and pressed
- 2 tablespoons olive oil
- 1/2 teaspoon basil
- 1/2 teaspoon oregano
- 1/4 teaspoon paprika
- 1/4 teaspoon cayenne pepper
- 1/4 teaspoon onion powder
- 1/4 teaspoon garlic powder
- Salt and pepper

Instructions

- Preheat oven to 375°.
- Mix olive oil and all the herbs and spices.
- Slice tofu into long strips, about 1/4 - 1/2" thick. Coat with marinade.
- Place strips on a parchment paper lined baking sheet, and bake at 375° for 20 minutes. Flip, and bake another 15-20 minutes, or until crispy on the outside.

Nutrition Facts

Baked Tofu Fries

Calories 132 Calories from Fat 90

Total Fat 10g 15%

Saturated Fat 1g 5%

Cholesterol 0mg 0%

Hemp Seed Cauliflower Rice Pilaf

Prep Time 5 minutes
Cook Time 5 minutes
Total Time 10 minutes
Calories 208 kcal

Ingredients

- 1/2 head of cauliflower (2 cups cauliflower rice)
- 1/2 cup hemp seeds
- 4 pitted dates chopped - I used Deglet*
- 1/2 teaspoon turmeric
- 1/2 teaspoon cumin
- 1/2 low sodium vegetable broth
- 1/4 cup sliced almonds
- Salt and pepper

Instructions

- If you are using a head of cauliflower, cut it into large chunks and place in the food processor. Mix until it resembles a rice consistency.
- Place cauliflower rice in a pan along with hemp seeds, chopped dates, turmeric, cumin, vegetable broth, and salt and pepper. Cook until liquid is absorbed, about 5 minutes. Add sliced almonds.

Recipe Notes

If you are on a keto diet, you may want to use less dates, or omit them altogether.

Nutrition Facts

Calories 208 Calories from Fat 126
Total Fat 14g 22%
Saturated Fat 1g 5%
Cholesterol 0mg 0%
Sodium 5mg 0%
Potassium 133mg 4%

Ginger Sesame Walnut and Hemp Seed Lettuce Wraps

Prep Time 10 minutes
Total Time 10 minutes
Servings
Calories 382 kcal

Ingredients

Sauce

- 2 tablespoons low sodium gluten free tamari
- 1 tablespoon maple syrup
- 1 teaspoon toasted sesame oil
- 2 tablespoons brown rice vinegar
- 1 tablespoon minced ginger

Filling

- 1 cup chopped walnuts
- 1/2 cup hemp seeds
- 2 dates chopped
- 1/2 cup chopped cucumber
- 1/4 cup chopped carrots
- lettuce leaves
- sesame seeds optional

Instructions

- Mix sauce ingredients.
- Add chopped walnuts, hemp seeds, dates, cucumber, and carrots. Let sit in the fridge for at least an hour for the ingredients to combine.
- Pile mixture into lettuce leaves. Top with sesame seeds, if desired.

Nutrition Facts
Calories 382 Calories from Fat 279
Total Fat 31g 48%
Saturated Fat 2g 10%
Cholesterol 0mg 0%
Sodium 510mg 21%
Potassium 230mg 7%
Total Carbohydrates 13g

Sriracha Deviled Avocados

Prep Time 5 minutes
Total Time 5 minutes
Servings small avocados (or 2 large)
Calories 399 kcal

Ingredients

- 4 small avocados, halved and pitted (or 2 large)

Sriracha Filling

- 2 tablespoons vegan mayo
- 1/2 cup + 2 tablespoons avocado
- 4 teaspoons lime juice
- 2 tablespoons sriracha or more if you it really spicy
- 2 pinches chili powder
- salt and pepper
- paprika and cilantro for garnish

Instructions

- Mash all sriracha filling ingredients together until smooth.

- Fill the halved and pitted avocados with the deviled sriracha mixture and sprinkle paprika and cilantro on top.

Nutrition Facts

Calories 399 Calories from Fat 324

Total Fat 36g 55%

Saturated Fat 5g 25%

Cholesterol 0mg 0%

Sodium 235mg 10%

Potassium 1084mg 31%

Vegan Mashed Cauliflower with Caramelized Onions and Mushrooms

Prep Time 5 minutes
Cook Time 35 minutes
Total Time 40 minutes
Calories 56 kcal

Ingredients

- 1 head cauliflower chopped (2 cups)
- 1 tablespoon olive oil or Earth Balance
- 6 tablespoons unsweetened plain almond milk
- 1 onion chopped (2 cups)
- Salt and pepper
- Slash balsamic vinegar
- 1 cup sliced baby portobello mushrooms

Instructions

- Steam cauliflower. Set aside until cool. Mix in food processor with almond milk, salt, pepper, and olive oil or Earth Balance.
- Heat olive oil in a pan at medium low heat and add chopped onion. Stir the onion until it is coated with oil. Sprinkle a pinch of salt on the onions.
- Stir the onions every few minutes or so. Cooking will take about 20 minutes. Add balsamic vinegar to deglaze the pan after 15 minutes. Add sliced mushroom, and cook a few minutes more.

- Reheat mashed cauliflower on stovetop or in a microwave. Top with caramelized onions and mushrooms.

Nutrition Facts

Calories 56 Calories from Fat 27

Total Fat 3g 5%

Saturated Fat 0g 0%

Cholesterol 0mg 0%

Sodium 40mg 2%

Potassium 198mg 6%

Total Carbohydrates 4g

Mexican Cauliflower Rice

Prep Time 5 minutes
Cook Time 10 minutes
Total Time 15 minutes
Calories 28 kcal

Ingredients

- head of cauliflower approx. 8 cups, cut into large pieces
- 1 tablespoon olive oil
- 1/2 cup chopped onion
- cloves garlic minced
- tablespoons finely chopped serrano pepper
- 2 tablespoons tomato paste
- salt and pepper
- cilantro chopped
- limes

Instructions

- Put 1/2 the cauliflower in food processor and pulse until it resembles a rice consistency. Do the same with the other half.
- Warm olive oil in a large skillet over medium heat. Add chopped onion. Cook on medium heat until translucent.
- Add garlic and serrano pepper. Cook another minute longer.
- Add cauliflower, tomato paste, salt, and pepper. Cook until tender.
- Serve with chopped cilantro and limes.

Nutrition Facts

Calories 28 Calories from Fat 9
Total Fat 1g 2%
Saturated Fat 0g 0%
Cholesterol 0mg 0%
Sodium 36mg 2%
Potassium 106mg 3%

Tamari Seaweed Flax Crackers

Prep Time 5 minutes
dehydrate 1 day 4 hours
Total Time 5 minutes
Calories 30 kcal

Ingredients

- 1/2 cup flax seeds
- 1/2 cup golden flax seeds
- 1 1/2 cups water
- 2 tablespoon low sodium gluten free tamari
- 2 nori sheets broken up (1/2 cup)

Instructions

- Soak flaxseeds and tamari in water for at least an hour. Next, add nori. Mix thoroughly.
- Spoon 1 heaping tablespoonful per cracker on a Teflon sheet. Put in dehydrator and dehydrate at 110° for 24-28 hours, or until crispy. Turn over halfway through the dehydrating process so that they dehydrate faster.

Nutrition Facts

Calories 30 Calories from Fat 18
Total Fat 2g 3%
Saturated Fat 0g 0%
Cholesterol 0mg 0%
Sodium 69mg 3%
Potassium 48mg 1%
Total Carbohydrates 1g 0%

Sriracha Deviled Avocados

Prep Time 5 minutes
Total Time 5 minutes
Servings small avocados (or 2 large)
Calories 399 kcal

Ingredients

- 4 small avocados, halved and pitted (or 2 large)

Sriracha Filling

- 2 tablespoons vegan mayo
- 1/2 cup + 2 tablespoons avocado
- 4 teaspoons lime juice
- 2 tablespoons sriracha or more if you it really spicy
- 2 pinches chili powder
- salt and pepper
- paprika and cilantro for garnish

Instructions

- Mash all sriracha filling ingredients together until smooth.

- Fill the halved and pitted avocados with the deviled sriracha mixture and sprinkle paprika and cilantro on top.

Nutrition Facts

Calories 399 Calories from Fat 324
Total Fat 36g 55%
Saturated Fat 5g 25%
Cholesterol 0mg 0%
Sodium 235mg 10%

Vegan Pizza Football Cheese Ball

This Vegan Pizza Football Cheese Ball will be the hit of your Super Bowl party! It is easy to make, and sure to impress!

Prep Time 10 minutes
Total Time 10 minutes
Calories 94 kcal

Ingredients

- 1 (8 ounce) vegan cream cheese
- 1 (10 ounce) vegan mozzarella
- 1/4 cup sun-dried tomatoes
- 1/4 cup green olives
- 1 teaspoon basil
- 1 teaspoon oregano
- 1/2 teaspoon garlic powder
- 1/2 teaspoon onion powder
- 1 teaspoon red pepper flakes
- Salt and pepper
- 1/4 cup walnuts chopped (or other nuts)

Instructions

- Slice a small amount of vegan mozzarella off the block. Cut one long and four short strips of vegan cheese for the stripes on the football. Alternatively, you could make stripes using the vegan cream cheese.

- Mix all ingredients, except walnuts, in a food processor. Wrap vegan cheese ball in plastic wrap and let sit in the refrigerator for an hour.
- Form vegan cheese ball into a football shape. Coat in chopped walnuts. Add the stripes with vegan mozzarella or vegan cream cheese.

Nutrition Facts

Calories 94 Calories from Fat 63
Total Fat 7g 11%
Saturated Fat 2g 10%
Cholesterol 0mg 0%
Sodium 217mg 9%
Potassium 55mg 2%
Total Carbohydrates 5g

Chocolate Low Carb Vegan Fudge

This Chocolate Low Carb Vegan Fudge is melt in your mouth good! It only takes a few minutes to make with very few ingredients.

Prep Time 5 minutes
Total Time 5 minutes
Calories 97 kcal

Ingredients

- 1/2 cup cacao or cocoa powder
- 1/2 cup coconut oil melted
- 1/4 cup full fat coconut milk
- 1/2 teaspoon vanilla extract
- 1 teaspoon almond extract
- 2 teaspoons erythritol or 15-20 drops stevia
- pinch salt

Instructions

- If using erythritol, heat all ingredients in a double boiler or microwave until erythritol is dissolved. Mix all ingredients thoroughly.
- Fill either ice cube trays, muffin liners, or a plastic wrapped lined storage container. Refrigerate.
- Once cooled, if using the plastic wrapped lined container, pull fudge out and slice on a cutting board. Store in the fridge.

Recipe Notes

Nutrition facts are with erythritol, which contains 4 grams of carbs per teaspoon. So there's about 0.7 carbs in each piece of fudge, whereas stevia contains no carbs.

Nutrition Facts

Amount Per Serving
Calories 97 Calories from Fat 90
Total Fat 10g 15%
Saturated Fat 9g 45%
Cholesterol 0mg 0%
Sodium 1mg 0%
Potassium 64mg

Low Carb Vegan Almond Cookies

These healthy Low Carb Vegan Almond Cookies are a delicious low carb treat that you don't have to feel guilty about!

Prep Time 5 minutes
Cook Time 25 minutes
Total Time 30 minutes
Calories 87 kcal

Ingredients

- 1 cup almond flour super fine or the meal/ flour - both work
- 1 tablespoon flax meal
- 4 teaspoons erythritol
- 1 teaspoon baking powder
- 1/4 teaspoon salt
- 1/2 cup almond butter
- 1 teaspoon vanilla extract
- 1/2 teaspoon almond extract
- 1/2 cup unsweetened vanilla almond milk
- 4 teaspoons sliced almonds 2 per cookie

Instructions

- Preheat oven to 350°.

- Mix all dry ingredients. Add almond butter and wet ingredients.

- Mix thoroughly. Scoop tablespoonful sized balls onto a parchment paper lined baking sheet. Flatten and add two slivered almonds per cookie. Bake at 350° for 20-25 minutes or until golden.

Nutrition Facts

Calories 87 Calories from Fat 63
Total Fat 7g 11%
Saturated Fat 0g 0%
Cholesterol 0mg 0%
Sodium 42mg 2%
Potassium 83mg 2%
Total Carbohydrates 3g

Chocolate Coconut Almond Chia Pudding

This sweet Chocolate Coconut Almond Chia Pudding is made with rich coconut milk and layered with chocolate coconut almond butter.

Prep Time 5 minutes
Total Time 5 minutes
Calories 561 kcal

Ingredients

- 1/4 cup chia seeds
- 1 cup full fat coconut milk or unsweetened almond milk or a combination of the two
- 2 tablespoons cacao powder
- 1/2 teaspoon almond extract
- 1 teaspoon vanilla extract
- 1 tablespoon maple syrup or 10 drops stevia
- 2-3 tablespoons Chocolate Coconut Almond Butter*
- 2-3 tablespoons slivered almonds
- 2-3 tablespoons finely shredded coconut

Instructions

- Add coconut milk or almond milk to chia seeds. Let sit in the fridge for at least an hour.
- Add cacao powder, almond extract, vanilla extract, and maple syrup or stevia. Blend in a Nutribullet or food processor until smooth and creamy.

- Layer pudding with Chocolate Coconut Almond Butter, slivered almonds, and coconut flakes in dessert goblets or bowls.

Recipe Notes

For a vegan keto version omit the chocolate coconut almond butter, use very little, or replace the maple syrup with stevia in that recipe.

Nutrition Facts

Calories 561 Calories from Fat 432
Total Fat 48g 74%
Saturated Fat 26g 130%
Cholesterol 0mg 0%
Sodium 23mg

Neapolitan Chia Pudding

This healthy Neapolitan Chia Pudding can be eaten for breakfast or dessert. It is easy to make and great for on the go!

Prep Time 10 minutes
Total Time 10 minutes
Servings (8) ounce jars
Calories 277 kcal

Ingredients

Chocolate layer

- 2 tablespoons chia seeds
- 1/2 cup unsweetened chocolate or vanilla almond milk
- 2 teaspoons cacao or cocoa powder
- 1/2 teaspoon vanilla extract
- 1/4 teaspoon almond extract
- 8 drops stevia

Vanilla layer

- 2 tablespoons chia seeds
- 1/2 cup unsweetened vanilla almond milk
- 1/2 teaspoon vanilla extract
- 8 drops stevia

Strawberry layer

- 1/2 cup Strawberry Chia Jam
- 6 chopped strawberries
- 4 teaspoons cacao nibs

Instructions

- Chocolate layer: Mix chia seeds and almond milk. Let sit in the fridge for at least an hour. Mix in cacao powder, vanilla extract, almond extract, and stevia.

- Vanilla layer: Mix chia seeds and almond milk. Let sit in the fridge for at least an hour. Mix in vanilla extract and stevia.

- To assemble: Divide puddings between two 8 ounce mason jars. Layer into each 1/2 of the chocolate chia pudding, then 1/2 of the vanilla chia pudding. On top of the vanilla chia pudding layer 4 tablespoons Strawberry Chia Jam. Garnish with chopped strawberries and cacao nibs.

Nutrition Facts

Calories 277 Calories from Fat 108
Total Fat 12g 18%
Saturated Fat 2g 10%
Cholesterol 0mg 0%
Sodium 167mg 7%
Potassium 308mg

Pumpkin Chia Pudding

This smooth and creamy Pumpkin Chia Pudding is not only easy to make, but is healthy enough to be eaten for breakfast.

Prep Time 1 hour 5 minutes
Total Time 1 hour 5 minutes
Calories 138 kcal

Ingredients

- 1/4 cup chia seeds
- cup unsweetened vanilla almond milk
- 1 teaspoon vanilla extract
- 15-20 drops stevia or 2 dates softened in hot water
- 1/4 cup pumpkin puree
- 1/2 teaspoon pumpkin spice
- pinch salt
- chopped pecans

Instructions

- Mix chia seeds and almond milk. Let sit in the fridge for at least an hour.
- Add vanilla extract, stevia or dates, pumpkin puree, pumpkin spice, and salt.
- Mix in a high speed blender or Nutribullet until smooth and creamy. Garnish with chopped pecans.

Nutrition Facts

Calories 138 Calories from Fat 72
Total Fat 8g 12%
Saturated Fat 0g 0%
Cholesterol 0mg 0%
Sodium 167mg 7%
Potassium 149mg 4%
Total Carbohydrates

Keto Chicken Pot Pie

Cook Time22 mins
Course: Main Course
Servings: 8 servings
Calories: 297kcal

Ingredients

For the Chicken Pot Pie Filling:

- 2 tablespoons of butter
- 1/2 cup mixed veggies could also substitute green beans or broccoli
- 1/4 small onion diced
- 1/4 tsp pink salt
- 1/4 tsp pepper
- 2 garlic cloves minced
- 3/4 cup heavy whipping cream
- 1 cup chicken broth
- 1 tsp poultry seasoning
- 1/4 tsp rosemary
- pinch thyme
- 2 1/2 cups cooked chicken diced
- 1/4 tsp Xanthan Gum

For the crust:

- 4 1/2 tablespoons of butter melted and cooled
- 1/3 cup coconut flour

- 2 tablespoons full fat sour cream
- 4 eggs
- 1/4 teaspoon salt
- 1/4 teaspoon baking powder
- 1 1/3 cup sharp shredded cheddar cheese or mozzarella shredded

Instructions

- Cook 1 to 1 1/2 lbs chicken in the slow cooker for 3 hours on high or 6 hours on low.
- Preheat oven to 400 degrees.
- Sautee onion, mixed veggies, garlic cloves, salt, and pepper in 2 tablespoons butter in an oven safe skillet for approx 5 min or until onions are translucent.
- Add heavy whipping cream, chicken broth, poultry seasoning, thyme, and rosemary.
- Sprinkle Xanthan Gum on top and simmer for 5 minutes so that the sauce thickens. Make sure to simmer covered as the liquid will evaporate otherwise. You need a lot of liquid for this recipe, otherwise, it will be dry.
- Add diced chicken.
- Make the breading by combining melted butter (I cool mine by popping the bowl in the fridge for 5 min), eggs, salt, and sour cream in a bowl then whisk together.
- Add coconut flour and baking powder to the mixture and stir until combined.
- Stir in cheese.

- Drop batter by dollops on top of the chicken pot pie. Do not spread it out, as the coconut flour will absorb too much of the liquid.
- Bake in a 400-degree oven for 15-20 min.
- Set oven to broil and move chicken pot pie to top shelf. Broil for 1-2 minutes until bread topping is nicely browned.

Nutrition

Calories: 297kcal | Carbohydrates: 5.3g | Protein: 11.6g | Fat: 17g | Fiber: 2g

Easy Stir Fry Kimchi & Pork Belly

Stir-fry kimchi and bork belly is so simple to make yet out of this world satisfying! Dinner under 30 minutes, and Keto friendly.

Prep Time5 mins
Cook Time: 15 mins
Marinating: Time10 mins
Total Time: 20 mins
Servings: 3 people
Calories: 804 kcal

Ingredients

- 300 g naturally-raised pork belly
- 1 tbsp naturally-brewed tamari or soy sauce (gluten-free option: use tamari or gluten-free soy sauce)
- 1 tbsp naturally-brewed rice wine
- 1 lb kimchi (see notes below)
- 1 stalk green onion
- 1 tbsp sesame seeds (optional)

Instructions

- Slice the pork belly as thin as possible. Marinate in tamari/soy sauce and rice wine for about 10 minutes. If your kimchi isn't pre-cut, then cut into 1 inch size.

- Heat a heavy bottom pan (I use cast iron). While the pan is very hot, add the marinated pork belly, stir fry until nicely browned, for approximately 5 to 10 minutes. You should see some fat being cooked out of the pork belly at this point.

- Add the kimchi into the pan, stir-fry for another 2 minutes, for the flavour of kimchi and pork to completely mix.

- Turn off the heat. Thinly slice the green onion, and add to the stir fry.

- If available, sprinkle sesame seeds on top as garnish.

Recipe Notes

If you use a store-bought kimchi, make sure to check the ingredients. I use a home-made fermented kimchi that's free of MSG and added sugar.

CONCLUSION

The keto plan is a versatile and interesting way to lose weight, with lots of delicious food choices.

To thrive on the vegan diet, it is important to cover any nutrient deficiencies you may have from exclusively eating plant foods.

9 781794 180000